- Clinical Nutrition -

THERAPEUTIC FASTING AND UNLOADING DIET

Enteral and Parenteral Nutrition

FIRST EDITION

Dr. Amin Gasmi

© **Copyright 2020 by Dr. Amin Gasmi - All rights reserved.**

The contents of this book may not be reproduced, duplicated or transmitted without direct written permission from the author.

Under no circumstances will any legal responsibility or blame be held against the publisher for any reparation, damages, or monetary loss due to the information herein, either directly or indirectly.

Legal Notice:

This book is copyright protected. This is only for personal use. You cannot amend, distribute, sell, use, quote or paraphrase any part or the content within this book without the consent of the author.

Disclaimer Notice:

Please note the information contained within this document is for educational and entertainment purposes only. Every attempt has been made to provide accurate, up to date and reliable complete information. No warranties of any kind are expressed or implied. Readers acknowledge that the author is not engaging in the rendering of legal, financial, medical or professional advice. The content of this book has been derived from various sources. Please consult a licensed professional before attempting any techniques outlined in this book.

By reading this document, the reader agrees that under no circumstances is the author responsible for any losses, direct or indirect, which are incurred as a result of the use of information contained within this document, including, but not limited to, —errors, omissions, or inaccuracies.

DEDICATION

To the ultimate power of the universe, the power of love. For me, more than all: dad, mom, my wife, Alain, Cherif and Salva.

ACKNOWLEDGEMENT

I thank all those who throughout my life have contributed to my training and make me what I have become today: God, my family, my teachers, my colleagues, my friends, my students, my patients, my athletes, and everyone I have met on my way. I am also indebted to a large number of books and scientific articles, and I cannot thank their authors enough for their sharing and generosity.

TABLE OF CONTENTS

Dedication iii

Acknowledgement iv

1.0: Introduction 1

2.0: History of Fasting 4

3.0: Metabolism During Fasting 6

    3.1   Initial period of fasting - Period of emergency adaptation 8

    3.2   Second Period of Fasting 10

    3.3   Third "Terminal" Period of Fasting 12

4.0: Stages of Fasting Therapy 13

    4.1   Stages of the Unloading Period 13

    4.2   Stages of the Recovery Period 17

5.0: Dynamics of Laboratory Parameters During Fasting 19

6.0: Indications for Treatment by Therapeutic Fasting 21

7.0: Contraindications to Therapeutic Fasting 23

    7.1   Absolute Contraindications 23

    7.2   Relative Contraindications 24

8.0: Types of Therapeutic Fasting 26

9.0: Methodology of the Therapeutic Fasting 30

    9.1   Preparation Period 31

    9.2   Unloading Period (direct fasting) 32

    9.3   Recovery Period (exit from fasting or realization) 35

    9.3.1 Recovery period diet on juices after an unloading period of 7 days 39

    9.4   Possible Complications During Fasting and Prevention ... 44

    9.5   Indications for Stopping the Fasting 49

    9.6   Combining Fasting with Other Natural Approaches 50

10.0: Basics of the Unloading Diet Therapy 53

    10.1   Classification of Discharge Days 54

Author's presentation 61

References 62

INTRODUCTION 1

Therapeutic fasting and unloading diets are of considerable interest, both in the medical environment and in patients interested in natural and alternative methods of treatment. Therapeutic fasting is usually called unloading diet therapy since this approch includes not only fasting but also the recovery period, which is perhaps the most difficult stage for the patient and the doctor.

In recent decades, the number of patients with combined pathology has been steadily increasing. The life expectancy of people in developed countries is rising, and at the same time, the number of various pathologies increases with age. This leads to the need for the simultaneous administration of many drugs, which is accompanied by an increase in the number of complications of drug therapy, including allergic reactions, intolerance to drugs and a plethora of side effects. Often, there is also resistance to drug treatment.

These factors explain a large part of the interest of scientists and patients in the therapeutic fasting. The range of application of therapeutic fasting is extensive, and it can be used for combined pathology, providing a healing effect simultaneously on many organs and systems.

The therapeutic fasting is devoid of several significant drawbacks inherent in drug treatment methods, which is why it is especially indicated for patients who are resistant to certain drugs or with poor drug tolerance and allergic reactions.

With some diseases (some types of bronchial asthma, allergic dermatosis, psoriasis, hypertension, ankylosing spondylitis, etc.), the therapeutic effect of fasting is not inferior to the effect of drugs, i.e., the treatment method of choice.

Therapeutic fasting has a wide range of indications with a relatively small number of contraindications and has a beneficial effect on many concomitant diseases. It also helps to normalize metabolic processes and the function of the cardiovascular system, and as well improves the general condition of the patient. It is a powerful prophylactic, and normalizes the activity of the immune system.

The development of numerous modifications of therapeutic fasting makes it possible to individualize treatment taking into account the age, body weight, and mental status of the patient. Recently, special attention has been paid to the research for new modifications of therapeutic fasting and the possible combination of the method of therapeutic fasting with other non-drug approaches.

For all these advantages, therapeutic fasting is not a generally accepted and recognized treatment approach. In practical medicine and scientific circles, there are diametrically opposite views on therapeutic fasting. Two trends are clearly traced. Opponents of therapeutic fasting consider this treatment method not physiological, leading to severe biochemical changes in the body associated with metabolic disturbances. Proponents and propagandists of the method consider it universal, not bringing undesirable consequences to the human body.

Official traditional medicine recognizes today that the therapeutic fasting method can be effective in treating several diseases. However, therapeutic fasting is not a panacea for all diseases, and it is contraindicated for some patients.

Therapeutic fasting should be performed only in a hospital under the supervision of a specially trained doctor, otherwise, there is a real possibility of developing a variety of complications.

HISTORY OF FASTING

Fasting treatment was known since ancient times. It is mentioned in the writings and instructions of scientists from Egypt, India, China, Tibet, Scandinavia, Rome, etc. Famous thinkers, scientists of Pythagoras, Socrates, and Plato used fasting to improve mental activity and increase creative abilities. Fasting was prescribed by Avicenna to his patients. Hippocrates said "A man carries a doctor in himself, you just need to be able to help him in his work. If the body is not cleaned, the more you feed him, the more you will harm him. When the patient is fed too much, the disease is also fed. Remember - every surplus is contrary to nature. "

In the 19th century, many researchers in various countries studied the physiological effects of starvation. One of the founders of this method, Dr. E. Dewey, treated gastrointestinal diseases, obesity, depression, and other diseases with well-dosed and adapted fasting. His student and follower L. Butfield Hazard wrote the popular book, "Hunger - the cure for disease" She supplemented the Dewey method with the use of cleansing enemas, water procedures, massage, gymnastics, and recommended a vegetarian diet after fasting.

At the beginning of the 20th century, starvation propagandists were E. Sinclair, A. Suvorin, and other prominent figures of art, literature, and scientists. There is even more widespread therapeutic starvation with the emergence in medicine of the so-called reformist movement, which paid great attention to natural methods of therapy. In 1914, F. Segesser's book "Therapeutic Fasting" was published. Among the scientists involved in the fasting and unloading diet therapy, one can name a prominent pathophysiologist, rector of the Military Medical Academy in St. Petersburg, V. Pashutin, French doctor I. Vivini - the author of the acclaimed book "Treatment by fasting and natural methods". I. Vivini successfully used prolonged fasting for diseases of the cardiovascular system, liver, bronchial asthma, and allergic diseases.

The prominent advocate of fasting was Paul S. Bragg, and his work, "The Miracle of Fasting" became a bestseller for many years.

METABOLISM DURING FASTING

Hunger is a trigger for metabolic stress in humans. Under stress, secretion of adrenocorticotropic hormone, catecholamines, glucagon, glucocorticoids and vasopressin is enhanced. These hormones activate lipase and promote the flow of fat from adipose tissue into the blood in the form of free fatty acids. Free fatty acids circulating in the blood can provide the body with enough energy for a sufficiently long time (depending on the reserves of adipose tissue). With the massive entry of free fatty acids into the liver and their oxidation, a large amount of acetyl-coenzyme A is formed. However, the intake of acetyl-Co-A into the Krebs cycle is negligible. As a result, the liver begins to synthesize ketone bodies from acetyl-Co-A: acetone, acetoacetic and ß-hydroxybutyric acids. In this case, a compensated metabolic acidosis develops.

During fasting, blood glucose decreases, which leads to a decrease in insulin secretion, an increase in glucagon secretion, which stimulates the phosphorylase kinase in hepatocytes. This in turn, leads to the activation of phosphorylase and stimulation of glycogen breakdown with the formation of glucose. Thus, on the first day of fasting, the body is provided with energy at 80% due to carbohydrates and only 10-15% due to fats. After about 12-24 hours, glycogen stores in the liver and muscles are depleted. Hence, the energy needs of the liver and partially that of the muscles are satisfied by the oxidation of free fatty acids. On the 3rd day of fasting, the body receives 30–40% of energy from the oxidation of fats and 40–60% from carbohydrates.

Fasting leads to the excitement of the center of hunger in the hypothalamus. In the future, a high activity of the hunger center and low activity of the satiety center is maintained due to a decrease in the mass of adipose tissue and a reduction in the adipocyte production in the starving organism. The cause of this state is the effect of the anorexigenic hormone - cachexin, as well as the stimulator of satiety - leptin. Thus, the feeling of hunger persists for a significant part of the compensated period of fasting, then its intensity weakens, probably due to fatigue of the center or due to the production of anorexigenic cytokines.

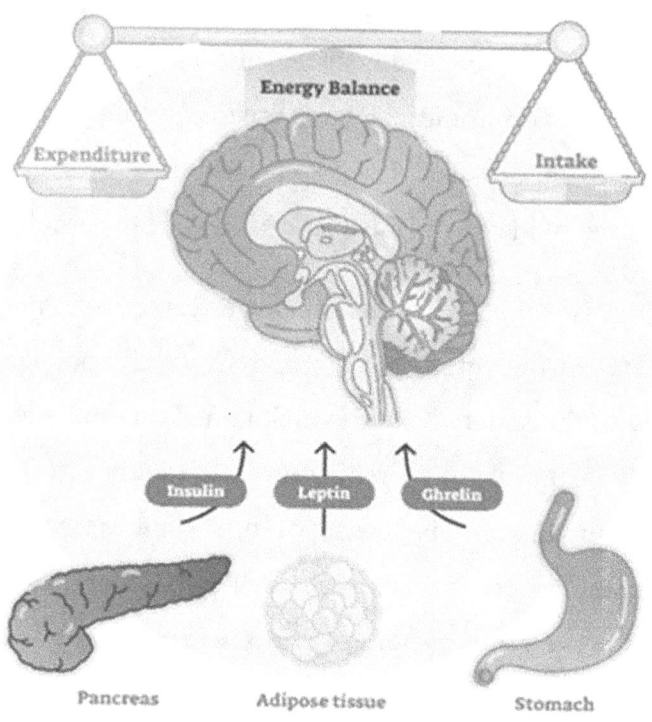

3.1 Initial period of fasting - Period of emergency adaptation

The period of emergency adaptation lasts from 2 to 7 days of fasting. On the 3rd – 7th day of fasting, stimulation of lipolysis and gluconeogenesis dominates. The brain in this period is still, as before starvation, able to use only glucose or glucogenic amino acids for energy needs. In order to provide energy to the brain, organs, and tissues that can directly use fatty acids and ketone bodies as fuel (heart, skeletal muscle, kidney cortex), the energetic metabolism switches to these products of lipolysis and conversion of ketogenic amino acids.

The initial period of emergency adaptation during fasting consists of the activation of glycogenolysis, the full use of carbohydrate reserves, and the stimulation of gluconeogenesis when transferring energy equivalents from the somatic compartment (adipose, connective tissue, and skeletal muscles) to the visceral one. This period cannot be characterized by the use of carbohydrates only or carbohydrates and fats since amino acids are utilized in gluconeogenesis. The mobilization of protein from the liver, blood, and gastrointestinal tract in the first week of fasting is even more active than from skeletal muscle. The proportion of calories derived from protein on the 2nd – 7th day of fasting increases to 8–11% versus 5% on the 1st day. It is due to the hormonal and metabolic changes described above during the first period of fasting that the main metabolism rises at the beginning of this period and then decreases progressively. Urea biosynthesis decreases, the proportion of non-urea nitrogen in the urine increases, and the production of uric acid in the tissues decreases. Significant accumulation of ketone bodies in the first days of fasting does not yet occur. Daily weight loss in the first period of fasting is maximum. If a normal adult man loses up to 3.1 g of nitrogen per day with urine (with feces up to 2.5 g and through the skin up to 0.5 g), then during the first period of fasting, nitrogen loss reaches 12 g/day, and then decrease by about half and stabilize at this level.

3.2 Second Period of Fasting

The second period of fasting begins with the second week of fasting. It has been proven that safe weight loss is 20–25%, in which case irreversible pathological changes do not occur in the tissues. When fasting for 25-30 days, weight loss is 12-18%, that is, below a safe norm.

The second period of fasting is the longest and determines the entire possible duration of fasting. The main thing that marks the beginning of the second period of fasting is a decrease in the use of amino acids for gluconeogenesis, an increase in the production and concentration of ketone bodies, and the beginning of the direct preferential use of ketones by the brain as fuel. At the same time, ketone bodies cover almost 70% of the energy needs of the brain. The rate of gluconeogenesis drops by 3-5 times; the daily loss of protein is stabilized, fat utilization continues at a high rate.

Hormonal changes characteristic of this period of fasting include a decrease in the production of stress hormones while maintaining a high glucagon-insulin ratio. An essential feature of endocrine-metabolic adaptation is a change in thyroid secretion. With starvation, thyroxine production and the conversion of thyroxine to highly active triiodothyronine are reduced. As a result, there is a decrease in the basal metabolic rate per unit of body weight by no less than 10%.

In the second period of fasting, there is a tendency for bradycardia, and respiratory rate decreases. In the kidneys, the sodium gradient decreases, and the ability to concentrate urine decreases, which leads to polyuria, which is typical for fasting. The gastrointestinal tract determines a decrease in peristalsis, which serves as one of the mechanisms of hunger constipation.

The general behavior of a starving person changes in the direction of less spontaneous activity, drowsiness, apathy, and a decrease in mental abilities; memory and attention develop. Resource-saving in the second period of fasting is expressed in a reduction in heat dissipation, relative ischemia of the skin develops, and its temperature drops, chilliness appears, and body temperature decreases to the lower limit of the norm.

In the second period, patients may experience headache, nausea, and weakness. Acidosis increases between the 6th and 10th day, after which an "acidotic crisis" occurs, and the patient's condition improves dramatically. Acidotic crisis arises as a result of the transition of the body to an endogenous diet, in which the heart and brain adapt to the satisfaction of a significant share of their energy requirements due to the oxidation of ketone bodies. Acidosis decreases, and the patient easily tolerates starvation. It is proved that during fasting, acidosis is compensated, and it is useful, as it promotes the fixation of blood-soluble carbon dioxide by the principle of photosynthesis. In this case, the disposal of ketone bodies is ahead of their accumulation.

During the first course of fasting, switching to the internal diet occurs on the 6–8th day, and in subsequent courses earlier, on the 3rd – 5th day. After the onset of the acidotic crisis, body weight in patients decreases significantly less during each following day.

After a properly conducted course of therapeutic fasting, mood improves, adaptation to stressful situations is restored.

3.3 Third "Terminal" Period of Fasting

Excessively long courses of therapeutic fasting (with a loss of body weight of more than 20–25%) can harm human health, since all fat reserves are depleted, and the body begins to expend vital proteins (especially the heart and brain), which leads to degeneration of internal organs and death.

The terminal period of decompensation during fasting corresponds to a loss of 40-50% of body weight with the loss of 100% of reserve fat and almost 97% of internal organ fat. It is characterized by an increased protein breakdown of the visceral compartment of the body. The excretion of urinary nitrogen increases due to non-urea fractions and due to urea. There is an increasing loss in the urine of amino acids, peptides, potassium, and phosphorus. Hyperuricemia and uraturia indicate the active decay of nucleoproteins. It increases slightly, per 1 kg of body weight, the main metabolism.

STAGES OF FASTING THERAPY

In the process of fasting, six stages of therapy are distinguished, which correspond to six clinical stages through which the patient successively passes through the treatment process - three on the unloading and three on the recovery period of treatment.

These stages correspond to physiological periods during fasting, both during the fasting phase and during the restoration and transition of the patient to adequate nutrition.

4.1 Stages of the Unloading Period

- **Stage of transition to endogenous nutrition;**

    At this stage, there are two clinical stages: stage I - the stage of nutritional arousal, the stage of anxiety and II - the stage of transition to endogenous nutrition, the stage of increasing ketoacidosis, the stage of "restructuring," switching.

- **Stage I - stage of food excitement, stage of anxiety;**

  Stage I usually lasts the first 2-4 days and is characterized by an increased feeling of hunger, headaches, "sucking" pains in the intestine; patients react sharply to the appearance and smell of food. Daily weight loss is 1-2 kg.

  In stage I, motor activity of the gastrointestinal tract periodically occurs, and the concentration of enzymes in the stomach and pancreas increases. Anaerobic decomposition of glycogen with the formation of glucose is activated. Glycolysis prevails in the first 16-18 hours of fasting.

- **Stage II - the stage of transition to endogenous nutrition, the stage of increasing ketoacidosis, the stage of "restructuring," switching.**

  After stage I, stage II begins — the transition to endogenous nutrition. At this time, a feeling of hunger is dulled, a smell from the mouth appears, the tongue is overlaid, moderate bradycardia, a decrease in blood pressure, stroke volume of the heart, and the occurrence of orthostatic reactions are noted.

  During this period, acidosis develops, associated with a drop in the alkaline reserve of blood and the accumulation of ketone bodies, which gradually increases, usually up to 7-9 days of fasting.

  Subsequently, within a day or even several hours, the phenomena of acidosis sharply weaken. This period was called the "acidotic peak" (F. Benedict, 1915).

In stage II, the body begins to function more economically, the main metabolism decreases (up to 30% of the initial), and the daily loss of body weight is 0.3-0.7 kg.

On the 6-8th day, the gastrointestinal tract stops functioning, and the so-called "spontaneous" gastric secretion appears. The secretion formed contains 25% of the protein, which is again absorbed. The body switches to endogenous nutrition, which produces endogenous saturation of the blood with nutrients, and the blood becomes "endogenously fed."

- **Stage of compensated endogenous nutrition;**

This stage corresponds to the III clinical stage - the stage of compensation, adaptation. The compensation stage lasts the first 15-20 days after the acidotic peak.

Ketonemia is reduced, and metabolic acidosis is compensated, which is manifested by an improvement in the patient's well-being, a decrease in feelings of weakness, hunger, and headaches. Patients increase their mood up to the development of euphoria; the symptoms of exacerbation of chronic diseases disappear or decrease. Daily weight loss is 0.2-0.5 kg. At this time, there is no significant change in the structures of the body, from 70 to 90% of the total energy consumption is provided due to the oxidation of triglycerides of fat depots and ketone bodies. There is a relative stabilization of metabolism, a decrease in the energy costs of the functions of physiological systems.

Approximately on the 20th day, a second acidotic peak occurs, similar in its clinical and paraclinical manifestations to the first, but less pronounced.

The stage of compensation continues to the physiologically acceptable level of expenditure of body resources. When resources are exhausted, the blood becomes "hungry" again, activating impulses appear, and a feeling of hunger (secondary food excitement) appears. The duration of this stage is a strictly individual indicator, which, on the one hand, depends on the defenses and compensatory capabilities of the body, and on the other hand, the duration and severity of the disease. The end of this stage is determined by some objective and subjective signs. The appearance of these signs corresponds to weight loss of 13-17% of the original.

- The appearance of increased appetite; increased feelings of hunger.

- Purification of the tongue from plaque up to its root.

- Reduced secretions with an enema (feces in the washings are practically not allocated, the liquid comes out transparent).

- The appearance of eye shine, blueness and purity of sclera.

- Persistent improvement in the clinical symptoms of existing diseases.

- The appearance of a "good color" face.

- Transition stage.

Following the stage of compensated endogenous nutrition of therapeutic fasting, a transitional stage lasts 1-2 days.

4.2 Stages of the Recovery Period

The period of exit from starvation, implementation, and preadaptation to endogenous nutrition.

- The stage of latent compensation of spent resources;

    At this stage, there are two clinical stages: I - asthenic and II - stage of intensive recovery.

- The asthenic stage ("growing food excitement against the background of irritable weakness," the stage of sensory-graded saturation) in most cases lasts 2-3 days. A feature of this stage is that, in a patient, saturation occurs very quickly after eating a small amount of food, but after 15-30 minutes, a feeling of hunger reappears. By the end of this stage, as a rule, there is an increased appetite.

- The stage of intensive recovery (secondary food stimulation, sensory-metabolic saturation) can last 5-7 days or more, depending on the duration of the unloading period. Satiety is held for 3-4 hours; the frequency of meals is reduced to 3-4 times a day. Appetite rises, which requires great care, patients begin to gain weight, normal regular stools are established, mood and well-being improve, physical strength is increased, and cheerfulness appears. There is a normalization of biochemical blood parameters.

- Hypercompensation phase of resources;

This stage corresponds to the III clinical stage - normalization.

The appetite becomes moderate, and the mood is even. Stage III is characterized by a complete restoration of all physiological functions of the body, stabilization of body weight.

During the process of resource overcompensation, the phenomenon of "activation" of metabolism and defenses is reliably revealed. This stage lasts up to 3-4 months, followed by the stabilization stage.

- Stage of stabilization;

In the process of this stage, the phenomenon of "tendency toward normalization" of higher nervous activity and metabolism is revealed.

DYNAMICS OF LABORATORY PARAMETERS DURING FASTING

- In the first days of abstinence from food, some patients have hyperbilirubinemia. By the time fasting ends, the serum bilirubin content is reduced and, as a rule, does not exceed normal limits.

- When fasting for more than two weeks, an increase in the activity of hepatic aminotransferase - AlAT is noted. A marked increase in the activity of AlAT by two times or more may indicate a violation of the integrity of the hepatocyte membranes and should serve as a signal to interrupt the unloading period.

- When fasting, the blood glucose level decreases.

- After a course of therapeutic fasting, a decrease in the content of cholesterol and triglycerides of blood serum is noted. With prolonged starvation, hypercholesterolemia is maintained, which may be an important factor in the pathogenesis of hungry hypertension in the period preceding serious alimentary dystrophy. Most likely, hypercholesterolemia also depends on increased excretion of VLDL by the liver, which receives a large lipid load during this period of fasting and, as far as possible, while maintaining balance, secretes VLDL, avoiding steatosis.

- With gout during fasting, the content of uric acid in the blood serum increases, which can contribute to the exacerbation of the disease.

- The protein-synthetic function of the liver can decrease only with prolonged periods of fasting.

- In a clinical blood test, as a rule, no significant changes are observed except a decrease in the hemoglobin content in individuals with iron deficiency.

INDICATIONS FOR TREATMENT BY THERAPEUTIC FASTING

- Hypertension I-II degree.

- Neurocirculatory dystonia in hypertonic and mixed type (the limitation is NCC in hypotonic type - there is the possibility of orthostatic collapse).

- Coronary heart disease, angina pectoris I, II, and III functional classes.

- Chronic obstructive bronchitis.

- Bronchial asthma.

- Sarcoidosis of the lungs stage I and II.

- Chronic gastritis with secretory insufficiency and hyperacid state, gastroduodenitis.

- Chronic non-calculous cholecystitis and pancreatitis.

- Biliary dyskinesia, irritable bowel syndrome).

- Diseases of the musculoskeletal system of inflammatory and dystrophic origin.

- Neuroendocrine disorders in chronic salpingo-ooparitis.

- Prostate adenoma.

- Alimentary-constitutional, diencephalic obesity.

- Resistance to drug therapy.

- Skin allergoses (chronic allergic dermatosis, neurodermatitis, psoriasis, eczema).

- Neuroses, depressive states, sluggish schizophrenia.

- Food and (or) drug allergy.

- Ankylosing spondylitis.

- Osteochondritis of the spine.

- Rheumatoid arthritis.

- Osteoarthritis.

CONTRAINDICATIONS TO THERAPEUTIC FASTING

7.1 Absolute Contraindications

- Severe deficiency of body weight (more than 15% of the proper values).

- Malignant tumors.

- Active tuberculosis of the lungs and other organs.

- Bronchiectasis disease.

- Systemic blood diseases.

- Type I diabetes.

- Thyrotoxicosis.

- Violations of the heart rhythm and (or) conduction of any genesis.

- Condition after a major focal myocardial infarction.

- Heart failure II B - III degree.

- Chronic hepatitis and cirrhosis.

- Chronic renal and renal failure of any genesis.

- Thrombophlebitis.

7.2 Relative Contraindications

- Coronary heart disease with rhythm disturbances and heart failure above stage II A.

- Severe hypotension.

- Cholelithiasis.

- Urolithiasis disease.

- Peptic ulcer of the stomach and duodenum.

- Chronic venous insufficiency.

- Type II diabetes mellitus.

- Gout.

- Febrile conditions.

- Pregnancy and lactation.

- Children's and senile age of patients.

- A particular problem is the use of therapeutic fasting in obesity. Despite the widespread use of therapeutic fasting in obesity, this method has several significant drawbacks, the main of which is the loss of muscle mass. However, the rapid loss of extra pounds is a powerful motivational factor for further work on the obesity treatment program.

- The list of indications and contraindications varies depending on the authors using the therapeutic fasting method. Diseases from the group of absolute contraindications move to the relative group, and then completely become indications for the use of fasting. All this is a matter of accumulating experience and the author's approach.

TYPES OF THERAPEUTIC FASTING

The following types of fasting are available:

- **Complete ("wet") therapeutic fasting;**

  The most common type of therapeutic fasting is complete fasting without the restriction of water intake.

- **Absolute ("dry") therapeutic fasting;**

  From a physiological point of view, the body does not experience a significant liquid deficiency during complete starvation. For every kilogram of fissile fat mass (or glycogen), up to 1 liter of endogenous (metabolic) water is released. The daily loss of body fluid through the skin, lungs, and kidneys is 1.5–2 L at normal ambient temperature. Thus, the water deficit does not exceed 0.5-1 liter per day, which is quite physiologically acceptable under conditions of reduced basic metabolism. Therefore, long periods of "dry" starvation lead to dehydration. If the absolute absence of water and food does not exceed 3-4 days, then the dehydration of the body does not go beyond a mild extent.

The positive aspects of short-term "dry" fasting are the reduction in the time of the onset of the stages of the unloading period. The stage of nutritional arousal lasts several hours, the stage of increasing ketoacidosis - from 1 to 3 days, "ketoacidotic crisis" (2–3 days later).

With this type of therapeutic fasting, a significant loss in body weight (2-3 kg/day) occurs, with 40% being in the water, 30-40% in fat, 15-20% in lean body mass, mainly liver and muscle glycogen.

In clinical practice, a short, 1-3 day absolute fasting is usually used. Laxatives and cleansing enemas before absolute fasting and during it are usually not prescribed.

"Dry" starvation, contrary to popular belief, is objectively tolerated easier than "wet." In many diseases (bronchial asthma, hypertension, allergoses, etc.), higher efficiency of "dry" 3-day fasting is shown in comparison with 3-day "wet" fasting. It can be considered that three days of absolute fasting correspond to 7-9 days of complete fasting without limitation of water.

"Dry" starvation is contraindicated in urolithiasis, cholelithiasis, thrombophlebitis and varicose veins, blood clotting disorders.

- **Combined (absolute and complete) therapeutic fasting;**

The methodology provides for the consistent use of 2-3-day absolute and 10-14-day complete therapeutic fasting.

With this technique, for 1-3 days (according to individual tolerance), patients are encouraged to refrain from eating food and water, cleansing enemas are not prescribed. Starting from 2-4 days, patients resume taking water, limiting it to 10-12 mg/kg of body weight per day for the entire unloading period, and continue complete fasting according to the usual therapeutic fasting technique.

A number of researchers note that the use of combined fasting allows you to achieve an earlier onset of an acidotic peak, a greater reduction in body fat mass. In the treatment of patients with arterial hypertension, normalization of blood pressure occurs earlier, which reduces the duration of the unloading period, and, accordingly, the duration of inpatient treatment of patients. The specified technique is the method of choice for complicating the underlying disease with obesity and edematous syndrome. In addition, the combination of dry and wet fasting is well tolerated by patients, has a therapeutic effect while reducing the overall duration of therapeutic fasting, and optimizes the timing of its conduct due to the earlier onset of an acidotic crisis.

- **Fractional fasting;**

  This type of fasting involves several (usually 3), repeated and following one after another cycle (fractions) of discharge periods. The average duration of the unloading period is 14 days, with an interval between cycles of 62 days; the total duration of treatment is 6 months. It is possible to use both full and combined therapeutic fasting.

- **Step therapeutic fasting;**

  Some fasting clinics proposed stepwise fasting for patients with obesity and poor tolerance of long periods of fasting. In this case, the patient is starving before the onset of the acidotic crisis (5–7 days), followed by a recovery period equal to half the fasting period, then again starvation before the crisis and a recovery period lasting half the fasting period. In total, 3-4 steps are carried out.

  The use of this technique is advisable for poor tolerance of long periods of fasting with hypertension, especially for patients older than 55 years. The technique may be the method of choice in patients with an increased risk intolerance to long discharge and fasting periods.

METHODOLOGY OF THE THERAPEUTIC FASTING

A dosed starvation method, and in subsequent years, significantly supplemented by other specialists in therapeutic fasting, consists in voluntary abstinence from eating with unlimited water and some detoxification hygiene procedures (water procedures, daily cleansing enemas, etc.) followed by restorative dietary nutrition according to a special scheme.

Unloading and dietary therapy should be carried out in specialized departments of the hospital or in medical institutions of the sanatorium type. Medical fasting with a period of unloading period of 14 days or more is recommended only in a specialized department of the hospital.

During the therapeutic fasting, the preparatory, unloading, and recovery periods are distinguished.

Their implementation is strictly regulated. Repeated therapeutic fasting courses may be given no earlier than 4-6 months later.

9.1 Preparation Period

At the prehospital stage, patients are selected taking into account indications and contraindications. In the preparatory period, individual and collective informational preparation of patients for this method of treatment is carried out, since the method of therapeutic fasting implies the active participation of the patient himself, and he should be familiar with the essence of the method, the timing, the main changes in the body during food deprivation, and the treatment regimen. It is necessary to coordinate with the patient the duration of the fasting period, to familiarize him with the rules of behavior during treatment.

All patients undergo a preliminary examination: a clinical blood test, urinalysis, feces for helminth eggs, Wasserman reaction, a blood test for sugar and alanine aminotransferase (AlAT), chest X-ray, ECG, and women are consulted by a gynecologist. If necessary, additional examination methods are prescribed: sputum culture for mycobacterium tuberculosis, stool culture for dysentery and typhoid parathyroid group, sigmoidoscopy, gastroduodenoscopy, etc. Prior to hospitalization, it is desirable to sanitize the foci of chronic infection.

To conduct fasting, separate chambers should be located away from the dining room.

Before treatment, a saline laxative is prescribed (40-60 g of magnesium sulfate of magnesium chloride). The intestines should be completely cleaned; otherwise, patients may experience headache, weakness, and dyspeptic symptoms.

After the preparatory period, true fasting begins.

9.2 Unloading Period (direct fasting)

The duration of fasting is dosed individually depending on age, initial body weight, and the patient's diseases.

In most cases, the course of fasting is from 7 to 21 days. As a rule, the therapeutic effect is achieved precisely with a given duration of the unloading period. For preventive purposes, one can recommend short-term fasting with the time of the unloading period from 3 to 7 days.

Throughout the unloading period, the principle of voluntariness must be maintained.

The treatment regimen is active - free or ward.

Throughout the unloading period, patients are advised to follow the daily regimen, in accordance with their age and existing diseases.

As a drink, patients use water (mineral, distilled, boiled, or spring), rosehip broth, water with lemon juice, slightly brewed green tea, and slightly alkaline water. Drinking is used without restriction - from 1 to 1.5 (sometimes more) liters per day, which provides detoxification of the body by maintaining adequate diuresis. In the presence of chilliness, water can be consumed in a warm form.

During fasting, the volume of medications stops or significantly decreases. In some cases (severe hypertension, hormone-dependent bronchial asthma, etc.), it is permissible to take reduced doses of medications within 3-7 days of the discharge period. To prevent hypertension, some clinicians recommend the use of antihypertensive drugs in the early days of fasting.

It is strictly forbidden to smoke or take alcoholic beverages during the entire unloading period.

During this period, the smell of some types of food can irritate patients, causing some aggressiveness.

A night's sleep should be at least 8-10 hours. Before going to bed, a warm shower is recommended. With severe dry skin, you can use hygienic creams. It is recommended to carry out a hygienic toilet of the oral cavity at least 2-3 times a day (brushing, removing plaque from the tongue).

In the presence of allergic diseases, do not wear synthetic clothing or use cosmetics and washing powders.

Patients should be warned about the need for a smooth, unsharp recovery from bed.

During the entire period of fasting, cleansing enemas are carried out with a total volume of 1.0-1.5 liters of water 1-2 times a day. Enema temperature corresponds to the patient's body temperature. For deep cleansing of the intestines and to enhance the cleansing effect, the method of hydrocolonotherapy can be used. At the end of washing, according to indications, herbal decoctions and bifid preparations can be introduced. The number of hydrotherapy procedures is from 1 to 3 times a week. It is recommended that one procedure be performed at the beginning of fasting and one after the onset of an acidotic peak.

Physiotherapy exercises, outdoor walks (at least 3-4 hours a day), water procedures (circular shower, Charcot's shower, salt-coniferous bathtubs, pool), massage, and other methods of physical treatment such as paraffin, electrosleep, mud therapy, etc., is recommended. The volume of physiotherapeutic treatment is determined strictly individually, taking into account the existing disease.

Sauna is carried out in the first days of fasting when orthostatic reactions are not yet expressed.

Patients are examined daily by a doctor; blood pressure and heart rate are measured. In the history of the disease, the dynamics of the condition of patients, their tolerance to therapeutic fasting, are noted.

With the appearance of nausea for a long time, frequent vomiting, headache, abdominal pain, the intake of hydrocarbonate mineral waters, and cleansing enemas with a 2% soda solution are indicated. Carrying out these procedures can improve the condition of patients. With the appearance of indomitable vomiting and electrolyte disorders, treatment with hunger must be stopped.

9.2.1 Regimen of the day during therapeutic fasting

All days go by one-day mode:

- Climb

- Measurement of blood pressure and heart rate

- Weighing

- Oral hygiene

- Cleansing enema

- Shower
- Massage
- Easy charging
- Rest - 1 hour
- Walk - 2 hours, as much as possible
- Rest - 1 hour
- Walk - 1.5 hours or more
- Rest - 1 hour
- Walk - 1.5 hours or more
- Recreation
- Oral hygiene
- Cleansing enema
- Bath
- Hang up

9.3 Recovery Period (exit from fasting or realization)

The recovery period is a crucial stage of the fasting, as a violation of the rules for its implementation can lead to severe complications. Cases of death in people who spent the recovery period without medical supervision are described.

The recovery period in duration should be equal to two-thirds of the unloading period or somewhat longer. In the first week that patients are in the hospital, they are discharged with an open sick leave under the supervision of a doctor until the end of the recovery period. Disability is determined by the doctor of the clinic individually, depending on the duration of fasting, the patient's well-being, data from control tests, and the nature of the patient's work.

When conducting fasting for therapeutic purposes in patients with chronic diseases, a sparing regimen with a restriction of motor activity is prescribed for the first 4-5 days of rehabilitation treatment. Gradually, the boundaries of the patient's motor activity expand depending on his well-being.

In the case of unloading and dietary therapy with a prophylactic and restorative goal for practically healthy people, the regimen is practically unchanged.

With the cessation of hunger, cleansing enemas, massage, all physiotherapeutic procedures are canceled. In the absence of an independent stool, an enema is prescribed for three days (it is possible with a decoction of laxative herbs) or herbal laxatives.

The recovery period is carried out to switch the patient's body from endogenous to exogenous nutrition. When leaving starvation, there is a need for an individual diet, taking into account the nosological form of the patient's disease, initial body weight, duration of the unloading period, and the moment of the onset of the ketoacidotic peak. The result of the program is a daily diet, a printed appointment sheet.

The basic principles of restorative nutrition are: physiological and adequate diet, gradual expansion of the diet, and the fragmentation of nutrition.

For the recovery period, various options for diets have been developed using juices, whey from yogurt, and cereals. It is optimal to use a vegetable-milk diet with strict gradualness of daily increase in nutrition, both in assortment and in the volume of foods and dishes, with a gradual decrease in the number of meals from 7-10 to 3-4 times a day.

In the early days of the recovery period, patients quickly feel full, even with a small amount of food. In such cases, this feeling of fullness should not be overcome, and it is not necessary to consume the entire portion of the proposed food. As a rule, after 1-2 hours, these individuals again have a feeling of hunger, which serves as the basis for the next intake of a serving of juice, kefir, etc.

At the first meals, the food concentration is low (the juice is diluted with water, the cereal broth is not saturated, etc.), with repeated meals, the food concentration gradually increases.

Often, juices are used when leaving fasting, with freshly prepared fruit or vegetable juices preferred. Most commonly, apple is used, less often peach, apricot, plum, pear, and quince juices. You should not use tomato juice rich in sodium ions because it often causes fluid retention in the body; grape - due to sugary taste and possible development of flatulence; chokeberry juice, which in many patients provokes nausea and vomiting. Citrus juices (lemon, tangerine, orange) are undesirable in the presence of allergic diseases. With increased secretion of the stomach, which is usually accompanied by heartburn, the juice should be diluted four times.

Patients suffering from diseases of the digestive system and food allergies are prescribed restorative nutrition using mucous broths and cereals.

During the entire course of treatment, and especially in the recovery period, it is necessary to control the water-salt metabolism. For this, patients measure the daily amount of drinking water and excreted urine; the data obtained are recorded in a self-observation diary. Normally, diuresis is 400 ml less than the liquid you drink. With edema, the amount of fluid drunk is regulated so that it is approximately equal to the diuresis of the previous day. This restriction of water allows you to get rid of edema within 1-3 days. Diuretic drugs cannot be used to avoid seizures caused by a violation of electrolyte metabolism. The most pronounced and difficult to eliminate edema occurs in diet violators (the use of salt).

When leaving starvation, a restorative diet is prescribed, a feature of which in the first days is the exclusion of salt and protein foods: legumes, eggs, mushrooms, fish, and meat from the diet.

9.3.1 Recovery period diet on juices after an unloading period of 7 days

- 1st day. During the day, the juice is diluted with water (1: 1), a total of 0.7-1.2 liters. The juice concentration increases by the end of the day, and water can be consumed between meals.

- 2nd day. Before lunch, pure juice, 2-3 meals, after dinner - fruits or vegetables, preferably in a grated form.

- 3rd day. Vegetable fruits. Porridge on water, bread, and dried fruits are introduced.

- 4th day. Boiled vegetables, fruits, vegetarian soups, and sunflower oil are added to the menu.

- 5th day. Sour-milk products (kefir, fermented baked milk, etc.) are added in small quantities.

- 6th day. Cheese, sour cream, and salt are introduced into the diet.

- 7th day. Add eggs and cottage cheese.

- After seven days of the recovery period, foods with a high protein content are gradually introduced into the diet, first fish, legumes, then poultry, and meat.

9.3.2 Option of restorative mixed diet after an unloading period of 7 days

Out of hunger is designed for seven days. The hours of eating are indicated tentatively and can shift in one direction or another, depending on the patient's regimen.

1st day;

- 9 hours: Oatmeal jelly at the rate of 1 tbsp. 1 Hercules, domestic production without food additives in 1 glass of water. Simmer for 10-15 minutes.

- 12 hours: Repeated intake of jelly.

- 15 hours: Acceptance of 50% juice, preferably freshly made from green apples or oranges or carrots or cabbage or tomatoes. Tomatoes can be used only in season and in the absence of diseases of the joints and spine. With increased secretion of the stomach, which is usually accompanied by heartburn, the juice should be diluted four times. It is acceptable to use store juices in the same assortment, juices from baby food that do not contain sugar or salt.

- 18 hours: Repeated intake of 50% juice.

- 21 hours: 0.5 cups of 50% juice.

2nd day;

- It is similar to the 1st day. Acceptance of the same juices, but already 75%. In diseases of the gastrointestinal tract, alternate 50% juice with oat jelly.

3rd day;

- 9 hours: In the absence of stool - take boiled water 2 hours before taking 6-7 berries of prunes. With restored bowel function, instead of prunes, grated carrots with 1 tablespoon are taken. 10% sour cream.

- 12 hours: One of the following fruits: a green apple, orange, 2 tangerines or 1 cup of berries of the season.

- 15 hours: 75% juice.

- 18 hours: Salad of cucumbers, lettuce, parsley, and dill. You can fill the salad with 1 tsp. of any vegetable oil.

- 21 hours: 0.5 cups of liquid with dried fruits to choose from: 1 tbsp. of raisins or 2 pcs. Of dried apricots or 2 pcs. of prunes.

4th day;

- 9 hours: Fat-free or low-fat liquid sour-milk product, preferably with "bio" crops: 1% "bio" kefir, low-fat yogurt.

- 12 hours: If during this period, the intestines function normalized, we recommend preparing vinaigrette: beets, carrots, 1 tbsp. of sauerkraut, a small amount of potatoes, dill, parsley, green peas, 1 tbsp. of vegetable oil. In the absence of a chair - broom salad: fresh, grated carrots and beets in one piece and three parts of finely chopped fresh cabbage, a quarter of a green apple, and 1 tbsp. of vegetable oil. The volume of salad to increase to 2 glasses.

- 15 hours: One of the following fruits: a green apple, orange, 2 tangerines or 1 cup of berries of the season.

- 18 hours: Salad of cucumbers, lettuce, parsley, and dill. You can fill the salad with 1 tsp. of any vegetable oil.

- 21 hours: 0.5 cups of liquid with dried fruits to choose from: 1 tbsp. of raisins or 2 pcs. Of dried apricots or 2 pcs. of prunes.

5th day;

- 9 hours: 100 grams of dietary cottage cheese.

- 12 hours: Buckwheat porridge without the addition of milk and butter.

- 15 hours: Salad of cucumbers, lettuce, parsley, and dill. You can fill the salad with 1 tsp. of any vegetable oil.

- 18 hours: 100 g of grated cheese, white varieties, low in fat such as "Adygei" or soaked feta cheese or homemade cheese. Add up to 1 cup of finely chopped greens.

- 21 hours: 0.5 cups of liquid with dried fruits to choose from: 1 tbsp. of raisins or 2 pcs. of dried apricots or 2 pcs. Of prunes.

6th day;

- 9 hours: One soft-boiled egg with greens. With fibroids, replace the egg with dietary cottage cheese.

- 12 hours: One of the following fruits: a green apple, orange, 2 tangerines or 1 cup of berries of the season.

- 15 hours: Any vegetables, except boiled or stewed potatoes. You can use frozen mixtures of vegetables, cook a vegetarian soup.

- 18 hours: 100 g of non-oily fish with a calorie content not exceeding 40-50 kcal. Any preparation method other than toasting. Combine with a green salad.

- 21 hours: 0.5 cups of liquid with dried fruits to choose from: 1 tbsp. of raisins or 2 pcs. Of dried apricots or 2 pcs. of prunes.

7th day;

- 9 hours: Liquid fermented milk product in the form of yogurt or 1% kefir.

- 12 hours: Salad of cucumbers, lettuce, parsley, and dill. You can fill the salad with 1 tsp. of any vegetable oil.

- 15 hours: 100 g of chicken without fat and skin. Any method of cooking, except frying. Green salad.

- 18 hours: One of the following fruits: a green apple, orange, 2 tangerines or 1 cup of berries of the season.

- 21 hours: 0.5 cups of liquid with dried fruits to choose from: 1 tbsp. of raisins or 2 pcs. of dried apricots or 2 pcs. Of prunes.

9.4 Possible Complications During Fasting and Prevention

During therapeutic fasting, the development of certain complications is possible.

- Exacerbation of chronic foci of infection;

  With therapeutic fasting lasting more than two weeks, an exacerbation of chronic foci of infection is possible.

  It is assumed that after 15 days of the fasting period, most patients experience transient immunosuppression of all parts of the immune system. The clinical picture of the resulting exacerbation depends on the existing focus of infection (chronic tonsillitis, pyelonephritis, adnexitis) and general intoxication syndrome (fever, weakness, sweating, etc.).

In order to prevent exacerbation of infections, the following preventive measures are recommended:

- Exclusion of hypothermia.

- Compliance with an adequate drinking regimen (at least 1.5 liters).

- In the presence of chronic urinary tract infection, it is advisable to prescribe uroseptic herbal medicine.

- In the presence of chronic cholecystitis, it is advisable to conduct tububes two times a week.

- In the presence of chronic tonsillitis, daily (1 - 2 times a day) rinsing of the pharynx with a weak solution of potassium permanganate or furatsillin is recommended.

- In cases of the development of a pronounced exacerbation of chronic foci of infection, therapeutic fasting should be abolished, and restorative nutrition should be prescribed in combination with therapeutic measures aimed at treating the infection.

- Severe stage of increasing ketoacidosis;

In 3-5% of cases in the stage of increasing ketoacidosis, the following phenomena can be observed: debilitating nausea, repeated (up to indomitable) vomiting, cramping abdominal pain, and severe general weakness.

In these cases, they recommend the use of alkaline mineral waters or the intake of sodium bicarbonate of 2.0-3.0 g every 2-3 hours. With repeated vomiting, gastric lavage with a 3-5% sodium bicarbonate solution is recommended. In the absence of effect, repeated enemas with a solution of the same concentration and intravenous infusions of 300-500 ml of 5% soda solution are recommended.

In cases of indomitable vomiting, fasting is interrupted and restorative nutrition is prescribed. In some cases, with a persistent psychological orientation of the patient to treatment with hunger, the so-called "step" is allowed, when after 2-3 days of restorative nutrition, complete hunger is prescribed again. As a rule, with a repeated course, the stage of increasing ketoacidosis is easier for patients to tolerate.

The severe course of the stage of increasing acidosis is usually observed in patients suffering from chronic diseases for a long time, as well as in elderly patients when the crisis occurs on the 8-12th day of hunger.

- Orthostatic syncope (collapse);

    Patients prone to hypotension may experience an orthostatic reaction in the form of fainting (collapse). In this regard, patients should be warned about the need to get out of bed slowly, especially at night. They should avoid sudden movements. Smoking is strictly prohibited.

    In the event of a fainting condition, the following measures are applied: the patient is given a horizontal position with raised lower extremities, an influx of fresh air is provided, oxygen is inhaled, ammonia is inhaled, caffeine and cordiamine are administered. Medicines are administered in half dosage.

- Convulsive syndrome;

    In rare cases, with long periods of fasting (over 23-25 days), tonic convulsions of the finger, calf, and (or) chewing muscles may occur. This is usually due to shifts in water-salt metabolism. In such situations, it is sufficient to prescribe a 1% solution of sodium chloride in an amount of 150-200 ml inside. The salt solution is given in the form of heat 4-5 times a day.

- Renal colic;

Prevention of renal colic - compliance with an adequate drinking regimen. It requires drinking at least 1.5 liters per day and the use of hydrocarbonate mineral waters at the stage of increasing ketoacidosis. With the development of renal colic, generally accepted therapeutic measures are carried out: antispasmodics, anticholinergics, analgesics are prescribed, warmth on the lower back and/or a warm bath.

- Violation of heart rhythm and conduction;

This complication is rarely observed. More often, ventricular extrasystoles are observed.

In cases of development of cardiac arrhythmias, potassium preparations (panangin, aspartame, and other potassium preparations) and beta-blockers (obzidan or anaprilin, a quarter or half dose) are prescribed. In the absence of effect over the next 1-2 days, starvation is canceled, and restorative nutrition is prescribed in combination with the continued intake of potassium preparations.

- Acute erosive and ulcerative changes in the mucous membrane of the stomach and duodenum.

This complication is extremely rare. In the presence of acute erosive-ulcerative changes in the mucous membrane that appeared against the background of the fasting period, the fasting period is terminated, a restorative diet and appropriate drug therapy are prescribed.

- "Salt" edema;

"Salt" edema can occur in the recovery period of therapeutic fasting if the prescribed diet is not followed and premature consumption of sodium chloride. Violation of the diet can be manifested not only when the patients use table salt directly but also when it is orally administered with food (brown bread, salted butter, cheese, etc.)

The appearance of edema is accompanied by a feeling of heaviness in the head or headache, lethargy, decreased urine output, a significant increase in body weight during the day (up to 1.5-2 kg). In such cases, a salt-free diet is usually prescribed, and within 1-2 days, the edema disappears on its own. To accelerate the disappearance of edema, diuretics (kidney tea, hypothiazide) or laxatives (20-30 g of magnesium sulfate) are prescribed. Prevention consists of the exclusion of salt from the diet for the entire recovery period.

- Syndrome "food overload;"

It may occur in the first days of restorative nutrition if patients do not follow the prescribed diet, that is when overeating. Patients have a feeling of heaviness in the epigastrium, nausea, vomiting, and stool disorders. It is necessary to wash the stomach and take laxatives. After this, the patient is recommended to refrain from eating for one day. Preventive measures consist of strict adherence to the prescribed diet.

9.5 Indications for Stopping the Fasting

- The patient's categorical refusal to continue therapeutic fasting.
- Severe course of ketoacidosis, which cannot be managed by bicarbonates.
- Repeated orthostatic fainting or general weakness up to the development of adynamia.
- Persistent cardiac arrhythmias conduction.
- Increasing circulatory failure.
- Persistent sinus tachycardia (110-120 beats/min or more).
- Severe bradycardia (50 beats/min or less).
- Repeated attacks of hepatic and renal colic.
- An increase in serum aminotransferase activity and/or direct bilirubin content is two times higher than normal.

- Acute erosive and ulcerative changes in the mucous membrane of the stomach and duodenum.

- Weight loss of more than 15% of the original.

9.6 Combining Fasting with Other Natural Approaches

Many scientific studies indicate a significant increase in the effect of therapeutic fasting with the combined use of other non-drug methods.

- Acupuncture;

  Some specialists in therapeutic fasting indicate an increase in the therapeutic effect with a combination of therapeutic fasting and acupuncture.

  Reflexology is also effective in treating complications of therapeutic fasting.

- Homeopathic treatment;

  Homeopathic remedies are harmless and have no adverse reactions. This is important when combining homeopathy with healing fasting.

  In the preparatory and recovery periods of therapeutic fasting, any form of homeopathic medicine can be used.

  During the unloading period, the granules made on the basis of milk sugar used per os should be dissolved in cold water (at the rate of 8-10 granules per 50 ml of water), mix thoroughly after dissolution and take as prescribed. Other homeopathic dosage forms are recommended to be taken as usual.

- Physical therapy methods;

The methods of modern physiotherapy are very diverse, so they can be used not only to enhance the excretory and detoxification effect during therapeutic fasting (sauna, various water procedures, hydrocolonotherapy, etc.) but also to stop the exacerbation of chronic diseases during the unloading period (galvanization, pulsed electrotherapy, laser therapy, magnetotherapy, mud applications, etc.)

Physiotherapeutic procedures can significantly enhance the therapeutic effect of therapeutic fasting in chronic diseases.

- Phytotherapy;

There are published data on the successful use of herbal medicine for therapeutic fasting.

Decoctions of herbs are used as a washing liquid for cleansing enemas when rinsing the throat, for holding the tubub. Plant uroseptics are used to prevent urogenital infections during the discharge period. As a supportive therapy for diseases of the cardiovascular system during hunger, infusions and decoctions of herbs (motherwort, dill, valerian, chamomile, burdock, etc.) are prescribed.

- Tubation of the gallbladder, liver, and bile ducts;

Tubation is indicated in 90% of cases when, during an ultrasound examination, stagnation in the gallbladder and bile ducts is detected. A contraindication to holding tububes is the presence of large stones (more than 0.5-0.6 cm in diameter) in the gallbladder.

Before and after the tubing, an ultrasound scan is performed to identify contraindications and evaluate the effectiveness of the tubing.

Before tubage, it is advisable to cleanse the intestines with an enema.

On the day of the tube, the patient takes choleretic herbs (official collection No. 2 or collection No. 3) up to 500 ml. After that, the liver area is locally heated for 60 minutes. After 3-4 hours, a cleansing enema is done.

BASICS OF THE UNLOADING DIET THERAPY

During unloading days, voluminous, but low-calorie foods are consumed. Food is taken 5-6 times a day in equal portions throughout the day.

Calorie fasting days range from 600-1000 kcal.

On contrasting days, bread, everything sweet, and salt are excluded from consumption.

On an unloading day, the patient should not feel a strong feeling of hunger to avoid overeating in the following days.

Fasting days can be appointed on an outpatient basis for 1-2 days no more often than 1-2 times a week, and in stationary conditions, at the discretion of the attending physician.

10.1 Classification of Discharge Days

There are various options for unloading diets, which can occasionally be used or as part of various dietary programs to reduce the energy value of the daily diet or enrich it with some component or, for example, enhance the diuretic effect.

According to the predominance of food substances in diets, unloading diets are conventionally divided into protein (cottage cheese, meat, fish); carbohydrate (sugar, rice, and fruit); fatty (sour cream, cream); with the predominant use of liquids (juices, tea).

According to the prevailing food products, unloading diets are divided into vegetarian-only plant foods; dairy (milk, kefir, cottage cheese); sugar, meat, and fish; liquid (fruit and vegetable juices, rosehip broth, and mineral waters).

Special dietary magnesium and potassium (with increasing magnesium or potassium) diets and the Carrel diet are described separately by nutritionists.

10.1.1 Carbohydrate discharge diets

- **Sugar diet**

  Indications: acute nephritis, renal and liver failure, diseases of the biliary tract.

  Diet: 5 times a day for 1 cup of tea with 30 g of sugar.

- **Rice-compote diet (Kempner's diet)**

  Indications: arterial hypertension, circulatory failure, renal failure, liver, and biliary tract diseases.

Diet: 6 times a day, one glass of sweet compote, two times with sweet rice porridge, boiled in water without salt. Just a day - 1.5 kg of fresh or 240 g of dried fruit, 50 g of rice, 120 g of sugar, and 1.5 liters of liquid.

- **Apple diet**

Indications: obesity, arterial hypertension, circulatory failure, acute nephritis and renal failure, liver, and biliary tract disease.

Diet: 300 g of ripe, raw apples in raw form or the form of apple dishes, including baked apples 5-6 times a day, only 1.5-2 kg. 1.5 kg of apples - calorie content - 690 kcal. In chronic colitis with diarrhea, every 2.5-3 hours (5-6 times a day) is recommended; 250-300 g of mashed ripe apples without peel and seeds should be eaten.

- **Dried fruit diet**

Indications: arterial hypertension, circulatory failure, liver disease, and biliary tract.

Diet: 100 g of soaked prunes (dried apricots, raisins, etc.) 5 times a day, only 0.5 kg.

- **Watermelon diet**

Indications: arterial hypertension, circulatory failure, nephritis, gout, kidney stone disease without phosphaturia, liver, biliary tract disease, and obesity.

Diet: 300–400 g of watermelon pulp five times a day, only 1.5–2 kg. Additionally, liquid is not added to the diet.

- **Potato diet**

Indications: nephritis, arterial hypertension, and circulatory failure.

Diet: 300 g boiled in a peel or baked potato without table salt, only 1.5 kg.

- **Cucumber diet**

Indications: obesity, arterial hypertension, type II diabetes mellitus with obesity, nephritis, liver, and biliary tract diseases, gout, kidney stone disease without phosphaturia.

Diet: 300 g of fresh cucumbers without salt five times a day, only 1.5 kg.

- **Salad diet**

Indications: obesity, atherosclerosis, arterial hypertension, metabolic syndrome, nephritis, liver and biliary tract diseases, gout, kidney stones without phosphaturia, and uric acid diathesis.

Diet: In 1.2-1.5 kg of fresh vegetables and fruits that do not contain purine bases, add a small amount of sour cream or vegetable oil, 4-5 times a day, 200-250 g in the form of salads without salt.

- **Fruit and Egg Day**

  Indications: obesity. It is carried out with normal liver function.

  Diet: five times a day, one egg and 10 g of apples with a cup of broth of wild rose (without sugar). Calorie content - 650 kcal.

- **Oat diet**

  Indications: obesity, atherosclerosis with obesity. Diet: 140 g of oatmeal in the water five times a day, only 700 g of porridge (200 g of oatmeal); 1-2 cups of tea and broth of wild rose.

  200 g of oatmeal cooked in water - calorie content - 790 kcal.

10.1.2 Protein unloading diets

- **Milk (kefir) diet**

  Indications: obesity, atherosclerosis, arterial hypertension, metabolic syndrome, circulatory failure, nephritis, liver and biliary tract diseases, gout, and kidney stone disease without phosphaturia.

  Diet: 200-250 g of milk, kefir, yogurt (low fat can be) six times a day, a total of 1.2-1.5 liters. 1.5 liters of kefir - calories - 800 kcal.

  Milk diet option: every two hours, six times a day, give 100 ml of warm milk and at night 200 ml of fruit juice with 20 g of glucose or sugar. You can add two times a day, 25 g of dried wheat bread.

- **Curd diet**

    Indications: obesity, type II diabetes mellitus, atherosclerosis, and arterial hypertension with obesity, circulatory failure, liver, and biliary tract diseases.

    Diet: 70 g of cottage cheese 9% fat or non-greasy five times a day. Two cups of tea, one cup of broth of wild rose, two cups of low-fat kefir, only one liter.

    An option is the cottage cheese-kefir (milk) diet (Yarotsky's diet): 250-400 g of cottage cheese and 1 liter of kefir (milk) during the day.

    Reduced cottage cheese and kefir day: cottage cheese - 200 g, kefir - 400 g. Calorie content - 690 kcal.

    Variant of cottage cheese day: Cottage cheese with sour cream (400-600 g) or cheesecakes, pudding. Cottage cheese is divided into four doses of 100-150 g and 15 g of sour cream for each reception. In addition, they give two cups of coffee with milk without sugar and 1-2 cups of rosehip broth.

- **Meat (fish) diet**

    Indications: obesity, atherosclerosis, and metabolic syndrome.

    Diet: 70 g of lean boiled meat or boiled fish five times a day, a total of 350 g; 100–150 g of vegetables (cabbage, carrots, cucumbers, tomatoes) five times a day, only 0.6–0.9 kg; 1-2 cups of tea without sugar.

Option for meat day: boiled beef - 400 g, raw white and boiled cabbage - 400 g (or a salad of carrots, cucumbers, tomatoes, cauliflower). Two cups of coffee with milk without sugar, 1-2 cups of rosehip broth. Calorie content - 675 kcal.

10.1.3 Fat unloading diets

- **Sour cream (fat) diet**

    Indications: obesity, less commonly in type II diabetes mellitus with obesity.

    Diet: 80 g of sour cream 20% fat five times a day, a total of 400 g, 1-2 cups of wild rose broth.

- **Fatty day with cream**

    Indications: obesity.

    Diet: Cream 500-700 ml per day in equal portions every 2 hours in pure form or with coffee, tea without sugar.

10.1.4 Liquid unloading diets

- **Juice diet**

    Indications: obesity, atherosclerosis, arterial hypertension, type II diabetes mellitus with obesity, kidney, liver and biliary tract diseases, gout, kidney stone disease without phosphaturia.

    Diet: 600 ml of juice of vegetables or fruits, diluted with 200 ml of water or 0.8 l of rosehip broth, for four doses.

- **Tea diet**

Indications: acute gastritis, acute or exacerbation of chronic intestinal diseases with diarrhea.

Diet: seven times a day, 1 cup of tea with 10 g of sugar.

AUTHOR'S PRESENTATION

Dr. Amin Gasmi is an Algerian physiologist and orthomolecular nutritionist. He is currently the president of the Francophone Society of Nutritherapy and Applied Nutrigenetics. He is also the founder and managing editor of the International Journal of Integrative Physiology and Nutritional Sciences. He is a member of several international scientific organizations such as the International Society of Immunonutrition and the International Society of Orthomolecular Medicine. Dr. Gasmi has a multidisciplinary background and had the opportunity to work on several fields such as nutrition sciences, micronutrition, genetics, exercise physiology, applied psychology, physical therapy, physical training, and biochemistry. He has a triple competence of clinician through patients' and athletes' nutritional and physiological care, of scientist through his high quality published books and articles, and of professional trainer through the trainings and lectures he gives to medical doctors, health, and sports professionals.

REFERENCES

Casale J., Huecker M. R. (2020) Fasting. *StatPearls Publishing*

Harvie, M., & Howell, A. (2017). Potential Benefits and Harms of Intermittent Energy Restriction and Intermittent Fasting Amongst Obese, Overweight and Normal Weight Subjects-A Narrative Review of Human and Animal Evidence. *Behavioral sciences (Basel, Switzerland)*, 7(1), 4. https://doi.org/10.3390/bs7010004

Johnstone A. Fasting for weight loss: an effective strategy or latest dieting trend?. *Int J Obes (Lond)*. 2015;39(5):727-733. doi:10.1038/ijo.2014.214

Longo, V. D., & Panda, S. (2016). Fasting, Circadian Rhythms, and Time-Restricted Feeding in Healthy Lifespan. *Cell metabolism*, 23(6), 1048–1059. https://doi.org/10.1016/j.cmet.2016.06.001

Most, J., Tosti, V., Redman, L. M., & Fontana, L. (2017). Calorie restriction in humans: An update. *Ageing research reviews*, 39, 36–45. https://doi.org/10.1016/j.arr.2016.08.005

Redman, L. M., & Ravussin, E. (2011). Caloric restriction in humans: impact on physiological, psychological, and behavioral outcomes. *Antioxidants & redox signaling*, 14(2), 275–287. https://doi.org/10.1089/ars.2010.3253

Zubrzycki A, Cierpka-Kmiec K, Kmiec Z, Wronska A. (2018). The role of low-calorie diets and intermittent fasting in the treatment of obesity and type-2 diabetes. J Physiol Pharmacol. 69(5). https://doi.org/10.26402/jpp.2018.5.02

www.ingramcontent.com/pod-product-compliance
Lightning Source LLC
Chambersburg PA
CBHW070316220526
45465CB00004B/1872